EMERGENCY MEDICAL HANDBOOK

A Definitive Guide to Immediate Response for Common Ailments

Phillip J. Richmond

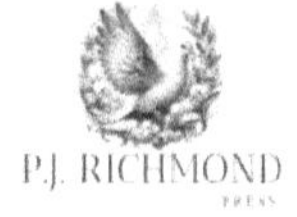

Dedication

To the unsung heroes of emergency care, whose quick thinking and unflinching devotion save lives every day. This book is dedicated to you, frontline responders, whose bravery and compassion make a difference in times of disaster. May this guide be a source of information and empowerment for you as you carry out your noble goal of providing instant assistance and comfort to people in need.

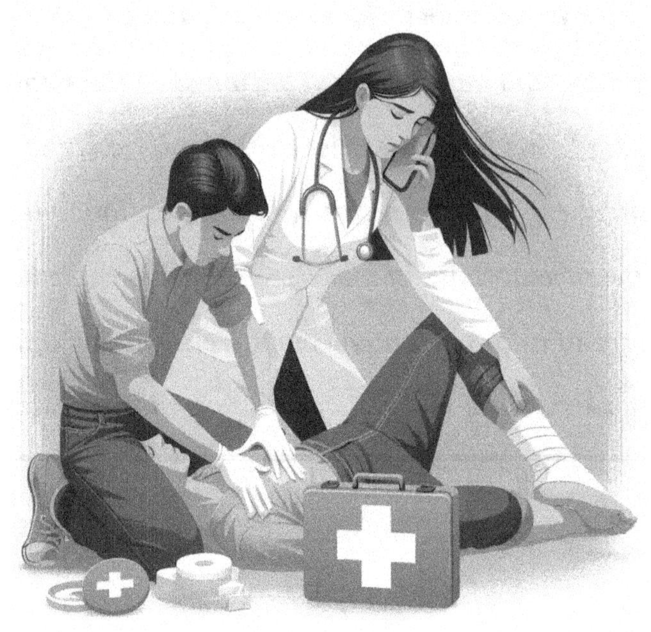

Table of Contents

Dedication 3

Introduction to First Response 7

1. Understanding the Basic First Aid Principles 11

2. Emergency Assessment and Response Procedures

.... 17

3. Cardiopulmonary Resuscitation (CPR) 23

4. Choking: A Lifesaving Guide to Quick

Intervention. 29

5. Seizures: Managing the Storm with

Compassion and Confidence 33

6. Allergic Reactions: Saving Lives with

Quick Intervention 39

7. Burns: Heal the Wounds with Knowledge

and Compassion 45

8. Bleeding: Mastering the Art of Quick Response 51

9. Fractures and Sprains: Managing Bone and Joint Injuries with Confidence 57

10. Heat and Cold Emergencies: Managing Extreme Temperatures with Care 63

11. Poisoning: Managing the Risks with Quick Action 69

12. Stroke: A Guide to Recognizing Symptoms and Responding Urgently 75

13. Heart Attack: A Comprehensive Guide on Recognizing and Responding with Urgency 81

14. Shock: A Comprehensive Guide to Understanding and Managing Critical Situations 85

15. Additional Resources and Training Opportunities: Enhancing Your First Aid Skills 91

Special Bonus 98

Introduction to First Response

Every instant matters in emergency medical care. Lives are on the line in the few seconds between crisis and resolution, and a first responder's quick actions can make the difference between life and death. This introduction welcomes you to the world of first response—a world where you have the ability to save lives. Consider this: you're traveling along a busy street, the bustle of city activity all around you, when suddenly, a cry for aid pierces the air. Without hesitation, you race to the scene, where you find a pedestrian wounded on the pavement. In that instant, the clock starts ticking—the golden window of opportunity during which your choices may make all the difference.

This incident exemplifies the significance of prompt and effective response in emergency circumstances. Whether it's a sudden cardiac arrest, a choking event, or a severe allergic response, the initial few minutes after an emergency are important. Every second that passes without assistance raises the possibility of permanent damage or perhaps death. But what does it mean to take prompt and effective action? It involves having the expertise and confidence to quickly analyze the situation, determine the most important requirements, and take decisive action to meet them. It entails knowing that even minor acts, when executed with precision and purpose, can have a significant influence on the outcome of an emergency.

It's normal to feel uneasy or afraid when confronted with turmoil and uncertainty. However, as a first responder, it is critical to develop a sense of confidence that allows you to remain cool and focused in the face of a disaster. Confidence is not acquired overnight; rather, it is cultivated through preparation, practice, and conviction in one's capacity to rise to the occasion when called upon. Building trust in emergency situations begins far before the crisis arises. It all starts with learning the information and abilities required to respond successfully to a variety of medical situations. You may build confidence in your abilities as a first responder by being familiar with fundamental first aid principles, learning CPR, and understanding how to spot and respond to common medical situations. But confidence is formed not only from technical expertise, but also from a genuine belief in your ability to make a difference. It's about following your intuition, capitalizing on your abilities, and accepting the challenge of becoming a ray of hope at someone's darkest hour. As you begin your path as a first responder, keep in mind that confidence is a mentality that you can grow and nurture day by day.

What exactly does it mean to be a first responder? Being a first responder is more than simply providing medical treatment; it is also about providing comfort, support, and reassurance during times of crisis. As a first responder, you play an important part in the chain of survival by bridging the gap between the time an emergency occurs and the arrival of expert medical assistance. Your position as a first responder is varied, with several tasks and duties. It entails analyzing the scene for any threats, assuring the safety of both oneself and the sufferer, and delivering rapid medical help based on the circumstances. It also requires good communication with bystanders, coordination with emergency services, and advocacy for the best possible outcome for the individual in need. But, perhaps most crucially, your duty as a first responder is based on compassion and understanding. It's about treating everyone you meet with dignity and respect, regardless of their situation. It's about making room for their concerns and anxieties but also providing a calming presence in the midst of chaos.

In the pages that follow, we'll go further into the complexities of first response, looking at the underlying principles that drive good emergency treatment. Together, we will learn how to negotiate the intricacies of medical crises with confidence, compassion, and an unrelenting commitment to people in need. Welcome to the realm of first reaction, where your actions have the potential to improve people's lives and make a long-term effect in the world. As we begin on this journey together, let us embrace the challenges that lie ahead, knowing that we can make a difference in someone's life when they need it the most.

Understanding the Basic First Aid Principles

Understanding and mastering fundamental first aid principles are critical components of efficient emergency medical treatment. From analyzing the scene for safety to administering life-saving methods such as CPR, these essential concepts serve as the foundation for all future activities. When confronted with a medical emergency, the ABCs of first aid serve as guiding principles, giving a methodical strategy to assessing and treating the most crucial components of patient care. Let us break out each component.

Airway: The first step in every emergency scenario is to check if the victim's airway is open and clear. A closed airway can quickly cause respiratory distress or even cardiac arrest, thus it is critical to respond fast. To evaluate the airway, gently tilt the victim's head back and elevate their chin to open it. Look, listen, and feel for indications of breathing, and if the airway is clogged, use the correct methods to free it, such as the head-tilt/chin-lift or jaw push technique. After the airway has been cleared, the next step is to examine the victim's breathing. Watch for chest rise and fall, listen for breath noises, and feel air movement on your cheek. If the person is not breathing or is having difficulty breathing, start rescue breathing by employing artificial ventilation procedures such mouth-to-mouth or mouth-to-mask resuscitation.

Circulation: After confirming that the victim's airway is open and breathing properly, the attention moves to checking circulation. Look for indicators of a pulse, such as a carotid pulse in the neck or a radial pulse in the wrist. If no pulse is discovered, immediately start chest compressions to keep blood flowing to essential organs. Remember to use the recommended compression-to-ventilation ratio for CPR (30 compressions to 2 breaths for adults) and keep going until aid comes or the sufferer shows signs of improvement.

Before providing help to a victim, it is critical to survey the scene for any risks that may jeopardize your or others' safety. This technique, known as scene safety assessment, entails evaluating the surroundings for any imminent threats, such as traffic, fire, or hazardous objects. By spending a few seconds to assess the situation before responding, you can reduce your risk of harm while increasing your efficacy as a first responder.

When evaluating the situation, keep the following aspects in mind:

- Look for any possible risks, such as downed power lines, leaking gas, or unstable structures.
- Scan the surroundings for signals of aggression or danger, such as the presence of weapons or hostile people.
- Consider using personal protective equipment (PPE), such as gloves or face masks, to protect yourself from bloodborne pathogens or other pollutants.
- Determine the best method for securely accessing the victim, taking into mind any hurdles or impediments that may prevent you from reaching them.

Remember that your safety is vital. If the situation is dangerous or you are unclear how to continue, wait for expert assistance to arrive before attempting to act. While knowledge is unquestionably important in emergency circumstances, it is hands-on training that puts theory into practice. Hands-on training allows you to practice and perfect your abilities in a controlled setting, ensuring that you are ready to respond confidently and successfully in a real-life situation.

There are a variety of ways to get hands-on training in first aid and emergency treatment, including:

1. **Formal training**: Enroll in a recognized first-aid or CPR course provided by organizations such as the American Red Cross or the American Heart Association. These courses often combine classroom education with hands-on skills training, allowing you to learn from skilled teachers while practicing on lifelike manikins.

2. **Community workshops**: Many community groups, fire agencies, and hospitals provide free or low-cost first aid and CPR training to the public. These courses offer a fantastic chance to learn fundamental life-saving methods while receiving hands-on training from local professionals.

3. **Simulation training**: Take part in simulation-based training exercises that mimic real-life emergency situations, allowing you to hone your abilities in a realistic and immersive setting. Simulation training can help you gain confidence in your talents and respond faster in high-pressure circumstances.

Whatever training method you pick, remember that practice makes perfect. The more you practice your abilities and get acquainted with emergency protocols, the more prepared you will be to respond efficiently when the occasion arises. Mastering fundamental first aid concepts is critical for everyone who wants to be a skilled and confident first responder. Mastering the ABCs of first aid, analyzing the scenario for safety, and participating in hands-on training will help you detect and respond to medical crises with more competence and precision. So, invest in your training, perfect your abilities, and empower yourself to help people in need.

The primary aims of first aid are to preserve life, prevent the condition from worsening, and promote recovery.

Emergency Assessment and Response Procedures

In the chaotic world of emergency medical treatment, the ability to remain cool under pressure can be the difference between life and death. As first responders, we are frequently pushed into chaotic and high-risk circumstances, where every choice we make can have far-reaching effects. In this chapter, we will look at the necessity of being cool under pressure, fast assessment strategies for swiftly evaluating patients, and how to prioritize activities in crucial situations to maximize patient outcomes.

In the midst of an emergency, it's normal to experience a rush of adrenaline rushing through your veins, increasing your senses and focusing your attention. However, instead of succumbing to panic or hesitation, that energy must be channeled into positive activity. Staying cool under pressure is not only a question of temperament; it is a talent that can be developed with practice, preparation, and a strong dedication to the work at hand.

One of the most effective strategies to remain cool under pressure is to create a routine or mental checklist on which you can rely in times of crisis. Breaking down big jobs into smaller, more manageable phases allows you to keep control and clarity even in the middle of turmoil. For example, in the event of a medical emergency, you may mentally rehearse the stages of the ABCs of first aid— Airway, Breathing, and Circulation—to ensure that no vital components of patient treatment are overlooked.

Another crucial part of remaining cool under pressure is the capacity to control your emotions and have a good attitude. Instead of obsessing on the seriousness of the situation or succumbing to feelings of dread or worry, concentrate on the work at hand and remind yourself of your qualifications and experience. Taking a proactive and solution-oriented attitude may instill confidence in people around you while also facilitating more efficient communication and collaboration during times of crisis.

In emergency medical care, timing is critical. Rapid assessment procedures enable first responders to swiftly acquire critical information about a patient's status, detect potentially life-threatening injuries or diseases, and implement necessary therapies promptly. While each scenario is unique, there are certain fundamental concepts and practices that may assist speed up the evaluation process and guarantee that no important facts are missing.

One of the most frequent fast assessment approaches is the "primary survey," which consists of a systematic examination of the patient's airway, breathing, circulation, disability, and exposure (ABCDE). Following this systematic method allows first responders to promptly identify and manage life-threatening situations in a rational and efficient manner.

Another useful fast assessment approach is the "focused assessment," which entails a targeted review of certain signs and symptoms relevant to the patient's principal complaint or presenting issue. This method enables first responders to focus on the most immediate issues while obtaining extra information to support their assessments and treatment recommendations. Regardless of the assessment approach used, first responders must be diligent and comprehensive in their examination of the patient's status. Pay close attention to vital indicators such as heart rate, blood pressure, respiratory rate, and oxygen saturation, and keep an eye out for any signs of deterioration or increasing symptoms that may suggest the need for immediate care.

In the fast-paced world of emergency medical treatment, the ability to prioritize actions properly is critical. When dealing with many duties and conflicting demands, it's critical to prioritize patients and therapies depending on the severity of their disease and the possible influence on patient outcomes. By using a systematic approach to prioritizing, first responders may guarantee that precious resources are deployed where they are most needed and that vital treatments are not delayed or neglected.

One often used technique of prioritization in emergency medical treatment is the "ABCDE approach," which entails putting patients into one of three priority categories based on the severity of their condition:

1. **Priority 1 (Immediate):** Patients with life-threatening injuries or diseases who require immediate medical attention to stabilize their condition and avoid further

deterioration. Examples include cardiac arrest, severe respiratory distress, and uncontrollable bleeding.

2. **Priority 2 (Urgent):** Patients with potentially significant injuries or diseases that require rapid medical treatment but are not life-threatening. Fractures, burns, and mild allergic responses are all possible examples.

3. **Priority 3 (Non-urgent)**: Patients who have minor injuries or diseases and may wait for medical attention without jeopardizing their health or well-being. Examples include small wounds and bruises, sprains, and low-grade fevers.

By classifying patients based on their priority level, first responders may better distribute resources and attention, ensuring that those in greatest need receive timely and appropriate care. Furthermore, selecting activities within each patient contact might assist first responders improve their efficiency and effectiveness by reducing time spent on non-essential tasks and increasing the impact of their treatments.

Finally, emergency assessment and response processes are essential to providing good prehospital treatment. First responders may improve patient outcomes and save lives in times of hardship by remaining cool under pressure, practicing fast assessment skills, and prioritizing actions in crucial situations. So, continue to believe in your training, trust your instincts, and never underestimate the importance of rapid thinking and immediate action when every second matters.

Cardiopulmonary Resuscitation (CPR)

Cardiopulmonary resuscitation (CPR) is one of the most important and possibly life-saving procedures in emergency medical care. CPR is a technique for maintaining blood circulation and oxygenation in people who are experiencing cardiac arrest or respiratory failure, boosting their chances of survival until more sophisticated medical care can be offered. Cardiopulmonary resuscitation (CPR) is a fundamental component of basic life support (BLS) and is intended to maintain essential functions in people suffering from cardiac arrest or respiratory failure. CPR is a mix of chest compressions and rescue breathing that aims to keep blood flowing and important organs oxygenated until more sophisticated medical procedures can be implemented.

The fundamental steps of CPR are:

1. **Evaluate the scenario for safety**: Before performing CPR, make sure that the situation is safe for both you and the victim. Look for potential risks, such as traffic, fire, or

electrical lines, and take the necessary procedures to reduce the chance of injury.

2. **Check for responsiveness**: Approach the person, gently shake their shoulders, and ask loudly, "Are you okay?" If the person does not reply or is not breathing properly, call emergency medical services (EMS) right away and start CPR.

3. Perform chest compressions by placing the person on their back on a solid surface and kneeling alongside them. Place the heel of one hand in the center of the victim's chest, between the nipples, and lock your fingers. With your arms straight, push forcefully down on the chest at a rate of 100 to 120 compressions per minute, allowing the chest to fully recoil between each compression.

4. **Give rescue breaths**: After every 30 compressions, open the victim's airway with the head-tilt/chin-lift or jaw thrust technique. Pinch the victim's nose closed and take two rescue breaths, keeping an eye out for a chest rise with each one. Continue with 30 compressions and two breaths until aid comes or the person shows signs of improvement.

Hands-only CPR, often known as compression-only CPR, is a simpler kind of CPR that focuses solely on chest compressions rather than rescue breaths. Hands-only CPR is advised for unskilled onlookers or those who are reluctant or unable to do rescue breathing, since it can still be helpful in restoring blood circulation and oxygenation in victims of sudden cardiac arrest.

The basic steps of hands-only CPR are:

1. Evaluate the scene for safety and responsiveness.

2. If the sufferer is unresponsive and not breathing regularly, contact EMS immediately and begin chest compressions.

3. Place the sufferer on their back on a sturdy surface, then kneel next them.

4. Place the heel of one hand in the center of the victim's chest, between the nipples, and interlock your fingers.

5. Press firmly down on the chest at a rate of 100 to 120 compressions per minute, allowing the chest to fully recoil between each compression.

6. Continue chest compressions until aid comes or the person shows signs of improvement.

Hands-only CPR is very successful when performed quickly by bystanders in the early aftermath of a cardiac arrest. By focusing primarily on chest compressions, bystanders may respond swiftly and give life-saving care without requiring considerable training or certification.

Automated external defibrillators (AEDs) are portable electronic devices that give an electric shock to the heart in the event of sudden cardiac arrest. AEDs are intended to evaluate the heart's rhythm and, if necessary, administer a shock, restoring normal cardiac function and boosting the probability of life. When used in concert with CPR, AEDs can greatly improve outcomes for those experiencing cardiac arrest.

The fundamental stages for utilizing an AED are:

1. Evaluate the scene for safety and responsiveness.

2. If the sufferer is unresponsive and not breathing regularly, call EMS right away and start CPR.

3. Locate the nearest AED and turn it on.

4. Follow the AED's visual and audio directions to place the electrode pads to the victim's chest and analyze their cardiac rhythm.

5. If the AED indicates a shock, make sure no one is touching the sufferer and hit the shock button as advised.

6. Resume CPR immediately after administering the shock, using the suggested compression-to-ventilation ratio, until rescue comes or the person shows signs of improvement.

AEDs are intended to be user-friendly and require little training to function properly. Communities can greatly increase survival rates for those who have sudden cardiac arrest by making AEDs more accessible in public settings and encouraging bystander usage.

Cardiopulmonary resuscitation (CPR) is a critical ability that can mean the difference between life and death in an emergency. First responders who understand the fundamentals of CPR, such as hands-only CPR and AED usage, can improve the chances of survival for patients of sudden cardiac arrest and respiratory failure. So, remember to remain cool, act decisively, and never underestimate the power of prompt action when every second matters.

CPR (Cardiopulmonary Resuscitation) is a crucial first aid skill used to revive an unconscious person whose breathing or heartbeat has stopped.

Choking: A Lifesaving Guide to Quick Intervention.

Choking is a terrible event that can happen abruptly and unexpectedly, posing a major threat to the victim's life if not treated swiftly. The first step in assisting someone who is choking is to identify the symptoms of choking. Common symptoms of choking include:

Symptoms may include difficulty breathing or speaking, gasping for air, throat clutching, and blue staining of the lips and fingernails. If you believe someone is choking, you must act swiftly since the airway obstruction can quickly lead to loss of consciousness and death if not treated immediately. If you see any of these indicators in someone, act quickly to save their life.

The Heimlich maneuver, commonly known as abdominal thrusts, is a technique for removing a blockage from the airway of a choking sufferer. It works by exerting pressure to the diaphragm, expelling air from the lungs to remove the blockage from the airway. Here's how to do the Heimlich technique to a cognizant choking victim:

1. Stand behind the choking sufferer and put your arms around their waistline.

2. Make a fist with one hand and press the thumb side on the victim's belly, somewhat above the navel but below the ribs.

3. Using your other hand, grip your fist and force inside and upward with a fast, upward thrust.

4. Repeat the thrusts until the impediment is removed and the person can breathe or cough normally.

The Heimlich technique must be performed with sufficient force to remove the blockage but not with such force that the person is injured. If the person loses consciousness while using the Heimlich technique, quickly drop them to the ground and start CPR. In addition to performing the Heimlich technique, it is critical to help both aware and unconscious choking sufferers. Here's how you can help aware choking victims:

1. Encourage the sufferer to cough aggressively in an effort to clear the impediment on their own.

2. If coughing is unsuccessful, do the Heimlich procedure described above until the blockage is removed.

If the person falls unconscious while choking, take the following actions to render assistance:

1. Take the person to the ground and immediately contact for emergency medical help.

2. Open the victim's airway with the head-tilt/chin-lift or jaw push method.

3. Look for evidence of breathing. If the sufferer is not breathing, perform CPR, beginning with chest compressions.

Continue doing CPR until emergency medical personnel arrive or the sufferer shows signs of improvement.

Choking is a potentially life-threatening situation that need prompt and deliberate intervention to avoid serious injury or death. Recognizing the indications of choking, executing the Heimlich technique, and administering aid to aware and unconscious victims can help you become a key lifeline for people in need. Remember to stay cool, respond fast, and put the choking victim's safety and well-being first.

Seizures: Managing the Storm with Compassion and Confidence

Seizures are a complicated and often terrifying medical phenomena that can strike abruptly and unexpectedly, leaving both the person experiencing the seizure and those observing it feeling overwhelmed and unsure. Seizures happen in a variety of types, each with its own set of symptoms and causes. Seizures are classified into two types: focal (also known as partial) and generalized. Within these categories, there are various varieties of seizures, each with its own set of qualities and characteristics. Below is an outline of the most prevalent forms of seizures:

1. **Focal seizures**: These occur in a single location of the brain and can affect only one section of the body or one side of the body. There are two forms of focal seizures:

- *Focal aware seizures (formerly known as simple partial seizures)*: These seizures may not affect awareness but may cause twitching, tingling, or sensory alterations in a single portion of the body.

- *Focal impaired awareness seizures (formerly known as complex partial seizures)*: These seizures entail a shift or loss of consciousness and might result in involuntary movements, bewilderment, or strange behaviors.

2. **Generalized seizures** are caused by aberrant electrical activity on both sides of the brain at the same time. Generalized seizures are classified into numerous subcategories, which include:

- *Absence seizures*: These seizures are usually seen in youngsters and are distinguished by a temporary loss of consciousness and blank gazing.
- *Tonic-clonic seizures*: Also known as grand mal seizures, these seizures include loss of consciousness, muscular rigidity (tonic phase), and rhythmic jerking motions (clonic phase).
- *Myoclonic seizures* are characterized by quick, short muscular jerks or twitches, which frequently occur in clusters.

- *Atonic seizures*, often known as drop attacks, involve an abrupt loss of muscular tone, which can lead to falls or drops without warning.

Understanding the various forms of seizures and their accompanying symptoms allows you to detect and respond to seizures in a more timely and appropriate manner, offering critical assistance to those suffering them.

Creating a safe environment during seizures is critical for reducing the risk of damage and ensuring the well-being of the person having the seizure. Here are some important actions to take to establish a safe atmosphere during seizures.

1. Remain calm and comfort the person having the seizure. Speak quietly and reassuringly, and let them know you're here to assist.

2. Remove any things or impediments in the near vicinity that might endanger the person during the seizure, such as sharp objects, furniture, or hot beverages.

3. If the person is seated or standing, gently lead them to the ground to avoid a fall or injury. Place a soft item or

pillow beneath their head to keep them from striking the ground.

4. Do not bind or keep the person down during the seizure, since this might result in damage or increased agitation. Allow the seizure to proceed while keeping a safe distance from the subject.

5. Once the seizure has ceased, assist the sufferer into a comfortable posture, such as on their side, to avoid choking or aspiration of saliva or vomit.

6. Stay with the person and offer comfort and support until they recover from the seizure. Offer to assist them with any immediate requirements, such as contacting a caregiver or providing medicine as needed.

Following a seizure, it is critical to give post-seizure care and support to assist the client in recovering and coping with the consequences. Here are some important measures to follow:

1. Stay with the person and carefully check their status when they recover consciousness. Look for symptoms of

damage or discomfort, such as disorientation, weakness, or trouble speaking.

2. Provide comfort and emotional support to the person while they recover from the seizure. Let them know you're here for them and that they're not alone.

3. If the client is disoriented or confused following the seizure, assist them in orienting themselves to their surroundings and offer mild reminders of what occurred.

4. Encourage the client to rest and relax for the rest of the day, particularly if they are exhausted or fatigued from the seizure.

5. If the person has a history of seizures or has had a lengthy or exceptionally severe seizure, encourage them to consult with their doctor for additional examination and treatment.

6. Offer to help the client with any practical requirements they may have, such as finding transportation home or calling a friend or family member for assistance.

Seizures are a complicated and frequently terrifying medical phenomena that needs rapid detection and adequate treatment. Understanding the various types of seizures, creating a safe environment during seizures, and providing post-seizure care and support can help you become a vital source of stability and reassurance for individuals living with seizures and their loved ones, allowing them to navigate the challenges of epilepsy with confidence and resilience.

Allergic Reactions: Saving Lives with Quick Intervention

Allergic responses can range from minor discomfort to life-threatening situations, therefore it is critical for people to be able to detect the symptoms and treat accordingly. Allergic responses occur when the immune system overreacts to a foreign material, known as an allergen, causing a series of symptoms. These symptoms might vary greatly depending on the degree of the response and the person's sensitivity to the allergen. Common indications of allergic responses are:

- Itchy and watery eyes.
- A runny or congested nose.
- Sneezing.
- Skin rash or hives.

Symptoms may include swelling of the face, lips, tongue, or throat; difficulty breathing or wheezing; nausea, vomiting, or diarrhea; and dizziness or lightheadedness.

It is critical to be watchful and proactive in diagnosing allergic responses, especially in those who have known allergies or a history of severe reactions. Early detection and care can help minimize the progression of symptoms and reduce the danger of anaphylaxis, a severe and sometimes fatal allergic reaction.

Epinephrine, which is often supplied by an auto-injector device such as the EpiPen, is the first-line therapy for severe allergic responses, including anaphylaxis. Epinephrine acts by swiftly constricting blood vessels and relaxing airway muscles, reversing the allergic reaction and restoring normal breathing and circulation. Here's how to give an epinephrine injection using an EpiPen:

1. Remove the EpiPen from its protective case and hold it firmly in your dominant hand, orange tip facing downward.

2. Pull the blue safety cap right off the top of the EpiPen. Do not touch the EpiPen's orange tip or black base, since this may mistakenly activate the injection.

3. Firmly press the EpiPen against the outer thigh of the person suffering the allergic response, ensuring that the

orange tip is pointing downward and the black base is in touch with the skin.

4. Swing the EpiPen forcefully and quickly into the thigh until you hear a click, indicating that the injection is initiated. Hold the EpiPen in place for several seconds to ensure that the entire dosage of epinephrine is administered.

5. Remove the EpiPen from the thigh and massage the injection site for 10 seconds to disseminate the medicine.

6. Dispose of the used EpiPen safely, according to the manufacturer's instructions and local medical waste disposal legislation.

It is critical to seek emergency medical attention immediately after giving epinephrine, as the medication's effects are transient and may wear off within a short period. Individuals who have received epinephrine should also be closely evaluated for evidence of repeated or worsening symptoms, which may need more doses or other measures.

Anaphylaxis is a severe, sometimes fatal allergic response that need prompt medical care. In addition to delivering epinephrine, there are numerous measures you may do to treat anaphylaxis and give crucial care to the person having the response. Here's what to do in case of an anaphylactic reaction:

1. Contact emergency medical services (EMS) right away and advise them that the person is having anaphylaxis.

2. Assist the patient in assuming a comfortable posture, such as resting flat on their back with their legs up, to promote circulation and respiration.

3. Keep a watchful eye on the individual for indications of respiratory distress, such as trouble breathing, wheezing, or cyanosis (bluish staining of the lips or fingernails).

4. If the person is cognizant and able to swallow, use antihistamines or other allergy drugs to assist relieve symptoms.

5. If the person's health worsens or they fall unconscious, do cardiopulmonary resuscitation (CPR) until aid comes.

6. Stay with the patient and offer comfort and support while they receive medical care for anaphylaxis. Offer to contact with healthcare providers and offer information about the

patient's medical history, allergies, and any drugs they are currently taking.

Allergic responses can pose serious hazards to people's health and well-being, therefore it's critical to be able to recognize the symptoms and respond appropriately. By acquiring the skills of delivering epinephrine injections and treating anaphylaxis, you may help save lives and promote safety in the event of an allergic emergency.

Recognizing the signs of allergic reactions, including anaphylaxis, and knowing how to administer epinephrine can be life-saving in severe allergic emergencies.

Burns: Heal the Wounds with Knowledge and Compassion

Burn injuries can range from slight pain to life-threatening crises, thus persons must be equipped with the knowledge and abilities to offer efficient first aid. A burn injury's severity is defined by a number of factors, including the depth and amount of tissue damage, the location of the burn, and the presence of aggravating factors such as age, pre-existing medical problems, and injury method. Burns are usually divided into three groups based on their depth and severity:

1. **Superficial (first-degree) burns**: These burns only affect the skin's surface layer, known as the epidermis. These burns are distinguished by redness, discomfort, and slight swelling, but no blisters or open sores. Superficial burns often heal on their own in a few days and seldom require medical intervention.

2. **Partial-thickness (second-degree) burns**: These burns cause damage to both the epidermis and the underlying

layer of skin, known as the dermis. These burns are distinguished by blistering, intense pain, redness, and swelling. Partial-thickness burns can take many weeks to heal and may need medical intervention to avoid infection and enhance healing.

3. **Third-degree burns (full thickness)**: Full-thickness burns penetrate all layers of the skin and may potentially affect underlying tissues like muscle, bone, or nerves. These burns are distinguished by white or burned skin, numbness or loss of feeling, and may seem leathery or waxy. Full-thickness burns require rapid medical treatment and may necessitate surgical intervention to heal the destroyed tissues.

When determining the severity of a burn injury, it's critical to evaluate the size and location of the burn, as well as any aggravating conditions like inhalation damage, electrical harm, or chemical exposure. Prompt evaluation and triage can assist ensure that people receive the right degree of care and support for their burn injuries.

Immediate treatment of burn injuries is crucial for reducing discomfort, avoiding more tissue damage, and accelerating recovery. Here are the most important measures to perform while administering first aid for burn injuries:

1. **Remove the source of the burn**: If the burn was produced by a heat source, such as fire or hot liquid, get the person away from the source of heat as soon and securely as possible. If the burn was produced by a chemical, thoroughly rinse the afflicted area with cold water to eliminate any leftover residue.

2. **Cool the burn**: Apply cool running water to the burnt region for 10 to 20 minutes to alleviate pain, edema, and tissue damage. Avoid using ice or ice water, since this can cause further harm to the skin and tissues.

3. **Protect the burn**: After the burn has cooled, use a clean, dry bandage to protect the wounded skin from additional harm and infection. Avoid applying sticky bandages or ointments to the burn, since they can trap heat and increase the risk of infection.

4. **Seek medical attention**: Depending on the degree of the burn damage, you may need to visit a doctor for additional examination and treatment. A healthcare practitioner should investigate burns that are partial or full thickness,

include sensitive areas such as the face, hands, feet, or genitals, or are caused by chemicals, electricity, or inhalation harm.

Once the initial first aid procedures have been implemented, it is critical to continuously monitor the burn damage and take precautions to avoid infection and promote recovery. Here are some crucial factors for treating burn injuries:

1. **Keep the burn clean and dry**: Do not touch or massage the burnt area, since this might increase the risk of infection. If the burn blisters or breaks open, carefully cleanse the area with gentle soap and water before applying a clean, dry bandage.

2. To protect the burn from additional harm, cover it with a clean, dry bandage to avoid friction, pressure, and infection. Avoid using sticky bandages or dressings directly to the burnt area, as this can aggravate discomfort and slow healing.

3. Keep an eye out for indications of infection, which include increasing pain, redness, swelling, warmth, or discharge from the burn site. If you feel that the burn is

infected, get medical help immediately for additional assessment and treatment.

4. **Follow medical advice**: If your burn damage necessitates medical treatment, carefully follow your healthcare provider's recommendations and attend all follow-up appointments as arranged. To improve healing and avoid problems, take any prescription drugs exactly as instructed and adhere to the recommended wound care techniques.

Burns are a common form of injury that need immediate and efficient first aid to alleviate pain, prevent complications, and encourage recovery. By assessing burn severity, offering timely care, and taking efforts to avoid infection and promote healing, you can help people recover from burn injuries and restore their health and well-being.

Basic wound care involves cleaning the wound with soap and water, applying an antiseptic, and covering it with a sterile bandage.

Bleeding: Mastering the Art of Quick Response

Bleeding situations can come suddenly and fast, therefore individuals must be prepared with the knowledge and abilities to appropriately manage bleeding. The first step in controlling external bleeding is to determine the severity of the hemorrhage and take prompt steps to stop it. External bleeding can be classified as arterial bleeding, venous hemorrhage, or capillary bleeding, with each needing a unique technique for optimal therapy.

1. **Arterial bleeding**: Arterial bleeding happens when an artery is cut or ruptured, causing brilliant crimson blood to erupt or pulse with every heartbeat. Arterial bleeding is the most serious form of bleeding and can be fatal if not treated quickly. To prevent arterial bleeding:

- Apply direct pressure to the wound with a clean cloth or sterile dressing, pushing hard to stop the flow of blood.

- If feasible, elevate the wounded limb above the level of the heart to limit blood flow to the affected area.

- If direct pressure and elevation are ineffective in stopping the bleeding, apply pressure on the closest pressure point between the cut and the heart, such as the brachial artery in the upper arm or the femoral artery in the groin.

2. **Venous bleeding** occurs when a vein is damaged, causing dark crimson or maroon blood to flow persistently from the site. Venous bleeding is less serious than arterial bleeding, but it still requires immediate treatment to avoid significant blood loss. To prevent venous bleeding:

- Apply direct pressure to the wound with a clean cloth or sterile dressing, pushing hard to encourage coagulation and minimize blood flow.

- If feasible, elevate the damaged limb above the heart level to limit blood flow and facilitate venous return.

3. **Capillary bleeding**: Capillary bleeding happens when tiny blood vessels near the skin's surface are injured,

causing blood to slowly ooze from the wound. Capillary hemorrhage is the least serious form of bleeding and may generally be treated with simple first-aid treatments. To prevent capillary bleeding:

- Using a clean towel or sterile bandage, apply direct pressure to the cut and keep tight for several minutes until bleeding stops.
- If possible, clean the wound with soap and water, then cover it with an adhesive bandage or sterile dressing to prevent contamination.

In severe or chronic bleeding, extra steps may be required to stop the bleeding and avoid future blood loss. When direct pressure alone is insufficient to control bleeding, pressure dressings and tourniquets are two viable options.

1. **Pressure dressings**: A pressure dressing is a bandage or dressing that maintains constant pressure on a wound, promoting coagulation and decreasing blood flow. How to apply a pressure dressing:

- Apply a clean cloth or sterile dressing directly to the wound and hold it in place with one hand.

- Wrap a bandage or elastic bandage tightly over the dressing and the damaged limb, providing enough pressure to limit the bleeding but not cutting off circulation.

- Use tape or fasteners to secure the bandage's ends so they do not come free.

2. **Tourniquets**: A tourniquet is a device that restricts blood flow to a limb, effectively cutting off circulation and preventing serious bleeding. Tourniquets should only be used as a last resort, when all other options have failed to stop the bleeding. How to apply a tourniquet:

- Position the tourniquet several inches above the wound, between it and the heart.

- Tighten the tourniquet until the bleeding stops, applying just enough pressure to prevent further harm.

- Secure the tourniquet and record the time it was placed, as tourniquets should not be left on for longer than two hours to avoid tissue damage and problems.

Internal bleeding occurs when blood seeps from injured blood arteries or organs within the body, which can lead to potentially fatal consequences if not detected and treated immediately. While internal bleeding is not always evident externally, there are various indications and symptoms to look for that may suggest internal bleeding, such as:

- Bruising or darkening of the skin around the injury site or elsewhere on the body.
- Abdominal discomfort or soreness, particularly if severe or chronic.
- Abdominal swelling or distention.
- Signs of shock include pale or clammy skin, a high heart rate, or low blood pressure.
- Dizziness, lightheadedness, or fainting.
- Blood in your urine, feces, or vomit.
- Breathing might be rapid or shallow.

If you believe that someone is having internal bleeding, get medical help right once for further assessment and treatment. Internal bleeding can be life-threatening and may necessitate surgical or other medical procedures to halt the bleeding and stabilize the patient's condition.

Finally, bleeding emergencies need early and efficient treatment to reduce blood loss, avoid complications, and improve recovery. By learning how to stop external bleeding, apply pressure dressings and tourniquets, and recognize indicators of internal bleeding, you may become an important first responder, helping to save lives and improve safety during bleeding crises.

Fractures and Sprains: Managing Bone and Joint Injuries with Confidence

Fractures and sprains are frequent injuries that can happen abruptly, causing discomfort and restricting movement. Fractures and sprains are both forms of musculoskeletal injuries, although they have distinct origins and features. Fractures are caused by the breaking or cracking of a bone, whereas sprains are caused by stretching or torn ligaments. Here's how to identify fractures and sprains:

1. **Fractures**: Fractures are divided into numerous categories, including:

- *Closed fractures*: The bone is shattered, but the skin is still intact.
- *Open fractures*: The bone breaks through the skin, creating an open wound.
- *Stress fractures*: Small cracks in the bone form as a result of repeated stress or misuse.

- Greenstick fractures: The bone bends and partially breaks, usually in youngsters with softer, more malleable bones.

Fractures may cause the following signs and symptoms:

- The wounded location is painful, swollen, and sensitive.
- A deformity or aberrant posture of the diseased limb or joint.
- Skin discolouration or bruises.
- Unable to bear weight or move the afflicted limb.
- Crepitus (a grating or grinding feeling) occurs when bone fragments scrape against one another.

2. **Sprains**: Sprains develop when a joint is stretched beyond its usual range of motion, injuring the ligaments that support it. Sprains may cause the following signs and symptoms:

- Pain, swelling, and soreness around the afflicted joint.
- Skin discolouration or bruises.
- The joint is unstable or loose.

- Difficulty bearing weight or engaging in routine activities.

To correctly diagnose fractures and sprains, a comprehensive physical examination is required, followed by imaging techniques such as X-rays or MRI scans to determine the degree of the injury.

Immobilization is an important aspect of treating fractures and sprains because it prevents additional harm and facilitates normal recovery. Immobilization procedures differ based on the kind and location of the injury, but may include:

1. **Splinting**: Splinting is attaching the wounded limb to a hard support, such as a splint or board, in order to immobilize the afflicted region and restrict movement. Splints can be made from cardboard, sticks, rolled-up towels, or commercially produced splints.

2. **Casting**: Casting is a more permanent method of immobilization that encases the wounded limb in a stiff plaster or fiberglass cast. Casting is often used to treat more

serious fractures or sprains that require prolonged immobility to heal correctly.

3. **Slinging**: A sling is used to immobilize and inhibit mobility in an injured arm or shoulder. Slings can be fashioned from triangular bandages or commercially available sling devices, and they should be adjusted to fit the damaged limb comfortably and securely.

When immobilizing a fracture or sprain, it is critical to ensure that the damaged limb or joint is properly aligned and that circulation is not disrupted. Check for numbness, tingling, or discolouration in the fingers or toes, which may indicate a lack of blood flow, and modify the splint or sling as needed to reduce pressure and improve circulation.

After the wounded person has been immobilized, it is critical to take them to a medical institution for further examination and treatment. When transferring wounded people, observe these measures to protect their safety and well-being.

1. **Stabilize the injury**: Before relocating the wounded person, make sure that the fracture or sprain is properly immobilized to avoid further harm during transport. Use

splints, slings, or other immobilization devices as needed to keep the damaged limb or joint in place.

2. **Support the damaged limb**: When helping the wounded person onto a vehicle or stretcher, make sure to support the afflicted limb or joint and avoid twisting or jarring motions that might worsen the injury. To offer support and comfort during transportation, use pillows, blankets, or cushions.

3. **Minimize movement**: Keep the wounded person as motionless as possible during transfer to avoid further harm or suffering. Avoid quick stops, starts, and sharp twists that may result in needless movement or jostling.

4. **Monitor vital signs**: During transportation, keep an eye on the wounded person's pulse, breathing, and state of consciousness. Be prepared to act quickly if there are any indicators of deterioration or discomfort.

5. **Communicate with emergency medical services**: If feasible, contact emergency medical services (EMS) while en route to the medical facility to give them with critical information regarding the type and severity of the injury. This will assist to guarantee that the wounded person receives the necessary amount of treatment upon arrival.

Fractures and sprains are frequent musculoskeletal injuries that require immediate and effective treatment to alleviate pain, avoid complications, and promote recovery. You may become a valuable first responder by learning how to recognize fractures and sprains, use immobilization methods, and transport wounded people securely.

Heat and Cold Emergencies: Managing Extreme Temperatures with Care

Extreme temperatures, whether blistering hot or deadly cold, can pose serious threats to people's health and safety. Heat exhaustion and heat stroke are two heat-related disorders that occur when the body's temperature cannot be efficiently regulated in hot and humid environments. While both diseases can be dangerous, heat stroke is a life-threatening emergency that needs prompt medical care. Here's how to identify and treat heat exhaustion and heat stroke:

1. Heat exhaustion is defined by excessive perspiration, dehydration, and overheating, which is frequently accompanied by symptoms such as:

- Excessive perspiration with pale, clammy skin.
- Tiredness, weakness, and dizziness.
- Nausea, vomiting, and diarrhea.
- Fainting, headache, or muscular cramps.

To treat heat exhaustion, take the person to a cooler, shady place and urge them to rest and rehydrate with cool water or sports drinks. Loosen tight clothes, administer cold compresses to the skin, and keep a watchful eye on the individual for any signs of increasing symptoms.

2. Heat stroke: Heat stroke is a medical emergency defined by a fast rise in body temperature, frequently reaching 104°F (40°C), associated with symptoms such as:

- Hot, dry skin that may seem red or flushed.
- Rapid, shallow breathing and a fast, weak pulse.
- Changed mental state, confusion, or loss of consciousness.
- Seizures or coma.

If you believe someone is suffering from heat stroke, call emergency medical services (EMS) right away and take urgent efforts to cool the person down while waiting for aid to come. Move them to a shady or air-conditioned environment, remove any unnecessary clothes, and administer cold water or ice packs to the skin to quickly reduce body temperature.

Hypothermia and frostbite are cold-related injuries that occur when the body loses more heat than it can create, resulting in dangerously low body temperatures and tissue damage. Here's how to diagnose and treat hypothermia and frostbite:

1. **Hypothermia**: Hypothermia is defined as a core body temperature below 95°F (35°C) with symptoms such as:

- Shivering, chilly, pale skin, and numbness.
- Drowsiness, confusion, or slurred speech.
- Weak, shallow breathing with a sluggish pulse.
- A lack of coordination or unconsciousness.

To treat hypothermia, relocate the person to a warm, covered location, remove any wet clothes, and wrap them in blankets or warm clothing to prevent additional heat loss. Provide warm, non-alcoholic liquids while constantly monitoring the individual for signs of improvement or worsening.

2. **Frostbite**: Frostbite occurs when the skin and underlying tissues freeze from extended exposure to low temperatures,

causing numbness, tingling, and tissue damage. Frostbite symptoms may include the following:

- Numbness, tingling, or pain in the afflicted region.
- White or grayish-yellow skin that is hard or waxy.
- Blisters or darkened, dead tissue in extreme instances.

To treat frostbite, gradually rewarm the damaged region by soaking it in warm (not hot) water or using warm compresses. Avoid rubbing or massaging the frostbitten region since it might cause more tissue injury. Severe or profound frostbite should be treated as soon as possible to avoid problems like infection or tissue loss.

Preventing heat and cold emergencies begins with taking proactive steps to protect yourself and others from excessive conditions when outdoors. Here are some important preventative tactics to keep in mind.

1. **Stay hydrated**: Drink lots of fluids, particularly water, before, during, and after physical activity, even if you don't feel thirsty. Avoid caffeinated or alcoholic beverages, since they might contribute to dehydration.

2. **Dress appropriately**: In hot weather, wear lightweight, breathable clothing to assist regulate body temperature and prevent sunburn. To remain warm and dry in chilly weather, layer your clothing and wear moisture-wicking textiles.

3. Take regular stops in shaded or air-conditioned spaces to relax, drink, and cool down when participating in outdoor activities in hot weather. In frigid weather, take pauses indoors to warm up and relax as necessary.

4. **Recognize the signs**: Familiarize yourself with the signs and symptoms of heat-related diseases like heat exhaustion and heat stroke, as well as cold-related ailments like hypothermia and frost bite. Stay watchful and ready to take immediate action if you or someone else exhibits indications of distress.

5. **Plan ahead**: Before engaging in outside activities, check the weather forecast and make adjustments to your plans to avoid high temperatures or poor weather. Bring water, sunscreen, hats, and gloves to keep safe and comfortable outside.

Heat and cold emergencies can pose substantial hazards to people's health and safety, but with adequate understanding and preparedness, they can be efficiently controlled and avoided. Stay safe and enjoy the great outdoors all year by identifying the indications of heat exhaustion and heat stroke, treating hypothermia and frostbite, and applying outdoor activity preventive methods.

Poisoning: Managing the Risks with Quick Action

Poison crises can occur suddenly, posing major threats to people's health and well-being. Household poisons may take many different forms, including cleaning goods, pharmaceuticals, plants, and chemicals. It is critical to be aware of potential sources of poisoning in the house and take preventative steps to avoid unintentional exposure. Here are some typical home toxins to look for:

1. *Cleaning products*: Bleach, ammonia, and drain cleaners can be toxic if consumed or breathed. Keep these goods out of reach of children and pets, and store them in their original containers with childproof lids.

2. *Drugs*: Prescription and over-the-counter drugs can be harmful if used incorrectly or in large quantities. Always follow the specified dose directions and keep drugs out of reach of children.

3. *Cosmetics and personal care products*: Items like nail polish remover, hair color, and mouthwash may contain

poisonous substances that, if consumed, might result in poisoning. Store these goods away from minors and use them according to the manufacturer's instructions.

4. *Plants*: Some common home plants, including lilies, oleander, and philodendron, can be deadly if consumed by humans or dogs. Learn to identify dangerous plants and avoid storing them in your house if you have small children or pets.

5. *Carbon monoxide*: A colorless and odorless gas created by faulty appliances such as furnaces, water heaters, and gas stoves. To avoid carbon monoxide poisoning, install carbon monoxide detectors around your house and get your appliances tested on a regular basis.

You may help decrease the danger of unintentional poisoning and keep your family safe by being aware of potential sources of poisoning in the house and taking precautions to avoid exposure.

In situations of suspected poisoning, prompt action is required to reduce the poison's effects and avoid additional injury. If someone has consumed a dangerous chemical, do the following steps:

1. ***Assess the problem***. Maintain composure and promptly analyze the individual's condition. Look for indicators of poisoning, such as nausea, vomiting, diarrhea, dizziness, trouble breathing, or changes in mental state.

2. ***Call for help***: If the individual is suffering severe symptoms or you are unclear of the toxicity of the substance consumed, contact emergency services (911) immediately for assistance. Give them as much information as possible regarding the poison consumed and the person's condition.

3. ***Contact poison control***: While you wait for emergency personnel to arrive, call your local poison control department for assistance and advice. Poison control professionals are accessible 24/7 to give expert assistance in situations of poisoning and can advise on the best course of action based on the type of poison consumed and the individual's symptoms.

4. ***Prevent future exposure***: If the poison was consumed orally, remove any residual poison from the individual's mouth and rinse it with water to dilute the poison and prevent additional absorption. If the poison was ingested,

place the person in a well-ventilated area and encourage them to breathe fresh air.

5. Stay with the individual and attentively check their condition while waiting for aid to come. Keep them quiet and comfortable, and be ready to provide first aid, such as CPR or rescue breathing, if required.

By acting quickly and decisively in situations of poison ingestion, you may assist reduce the poison's effects and secure the best possible outcome for the affected individual.

Poison control centers play an important role in handling poison crises, offering professional advice and support to both consumers and healthcare practitioners. Here's how to contact poison control in the event of a poisoning emergency.

1. ***Call the poison control hotline***: In the United States, the national poison control hotline is 1-800-222-1222. This hotline is maintained by qualified poison control professionals who can give quick aid and advise in the event of poisoning.

2. ***Offer information***: When calling poison control, be prepared to offer as much information as possible regarding the sort of poison eaten, the amount consumed, and the person's symptoms. This information will assist poison control personnel in determining the best course of action for handling the poisoning incident.

3. ***Follow instructions***: Poison control personnel are qualified to assess the degree of poisoning and give appropriate treatment and management advice. Prepare to follow up with healthcare providers or emergency services as necessary based on their suggestions.

4. ***Keep the hotline number handy***: Store the poison control hotline number on your phone or put it in a visible area in your house so that it is easily accessible in the event of an emergency. Share the number with family members, babysitters, and caretakers so that everyone understands how to get help in the event of a poisoning emergency.

In situations of poisoning, notifying poison control right away can provide you with expert information and assistance in managing the situation efficiently and ensuring the best possible outcome for the individual affected.

Poisoning crises can be terrifying and possibly fatal, but with the correct information and preparation, they can be efficiently controlled and avoided. Recognizing common home poisons, taking early action in situations of poison ingestion, and contacting poison control centers for information and support may help you become a critical first responder, reducing the consequences of poisoning and ensuring the well-being of people in need.

Stroke: A Guide to Recognizing Symptoms and Responding Urgently

Stroke is a medical emergency that demands prompt attention and action to avoid catastrophic consequences. A stroke happens when blood flow to the brain is disrupted or diminished, depriving brain cells of oxygen and nutrients. Several risk factors can raise a person's probability of having a stroke, including:

1. *High blood pressure*: Hypertension is the single most significant risk factor for stroke because it damages blood vessels and increases the likelihood of blood clots developing in the brain.

2. *Smoking*: Tobacco use, including smoking cigarettes or cigars and using smokeless tobacco products, considerably raises the risk of stroke owing to the damaging effects of nicotine and other substances on blood vessels and circulation.

3. *Diabetes*: People with diabetes are more likely to have a stroke because high blood sugar levels can damage blood vessels and raise the risk of atherosclerosis (artery hardening) and blood clots.

4. *High cholesterol*: Elevated cholesterol levels in the blood can cause plaque (fatty deposits) to form in the arteries, narrowing them and raising the risk of a stroke.

5. *Obesity*: Being overweight or obese raises the risk of stroke since it is linked to other risk factors such high blood pressure, diabetes, and high cholesterol.

6. *Physical inactivity*: A lack of regular physical exercise can lead to the development of other stroke risk factors such obesity, high blood pressure, and diabetes.

7. *Family history*: People with a family history of stroke or cardiovascular disease are more likely to have one themselves, because genetics can influence susceptibility to these disorders.

Understanding these risk factors and taking efforts to address modifiable risk factors such as high blood pressure, smoking, and physical inactivity can help people lower their chance of having a stroke and improve their overall health and well-being.

Recognizing the signs and symptoms of a stroke is critical for taking immediate action and seeking emergency medical attention. The F.A.S.T. acronym is a simple and effective method for recognizing stroke symptoms and responding quickly:

1. *Face drooping*: Have the person smile and see whether one side of their face droops or seems uneven.

2. *Arm weakness*: Have the person extend both arms and see whether one slips lower or is weaker than the other.

3. *Speech problem*: Ask the person to repeat a simple sentence while listening for slurred or garbled speech, difficulty speaking, or difficulty understanding words.

4. *When to call emergency services*: If you see any of these signs or symptoms, call 911 immediately and get medical assistance right away. In stroke treatment, time is of the importance, and every minute matters in terms of reducing brain damage and improving outcomes.

In addition to the F.A.S.T. evaluation, additional frequent stroke symptoms include sudden

- Numbness or weakness in the face, arms, or legs, often on one side of the body.
- Confusion, difficulty speaking or comprehending speech.
- Trouble seeing in one or both eyes.
- Severe headache without a known reason.

When a stroke is suspected, it is critical to seek emergency medical attention right once to limit brain damage and improve outcomes. Emergency medical therapy for stroke sufferers may involve the following:

1. ***Using clot-busting medicine***: If the stroke is caused by a blood clot that is preventing blood flow to the brain (ischemic stroke), clot-busting medication, such as tissue plasminogen activator (tPA), may be given intravenously to dissolve the clot and restore blood flow.

2. ***Endovascular therapy***: In some circumstances, a catheter-based method can be used to remove the clot directly from the blocked blood artery.

3. ***Managing consequences***: Stroke patients may require supportive treatment to treat problems such as high blood pressure, seizures, or brain swelling (cerebral edema).

4. ***Rehabilitation***: After the initial phase of treatment, stroke survivors may benefit from rehabilitation therapy to reclaim lost function and enhance their quality of life. Rehabilitation may involve physical therapy, occupational therapy, speech therapy, and other therapies suited to the individual's requirements.

Stroke sufferers can improve their chances of recovery and reduce long-term impairment by seeking emergency medical care as soon as possible and following through on appropriate therapies and therapy. Stroke is a medical emergency that needs quick attention and effort to mitigate its deadly effects. Individuals may become critical first responders by identifying stroke risk factors, executing an F.A.S.T. evaluation for stroke symptoms, and beginning emergency medical care as soon as possible, so saving lives and reducing the long-term burden of stroke on individuals and families.

Learning first aid can empower individuals to take immediate action in emergencies, potentially saving lives in critical situations.

Heart Attack: A Comprehensive Guide on Recognizing and Responding with Urgency

A heart attack is a life-threatening medical emergency that necessitates prompt treatment and intervention to reduce heart damage and improve outcomes. Heart attack symptoms can vary greatly from person to person and even between men and women. However, there are some typical indications and symptoms that may signal a heart attack is developing. These include:

1. Chest pain or discomfort is the most prevalent sign of a heart attack, and it might feel like pressure, tightness, squeezing, or burning in the chest. The discomfort might also spread to the arms, shoulders, neck, jaw, back, and belly.

2. ***Shortness of breath***: During a heart attack, you may experience difficulty breathing or shortness of breath, which is frequently accompanied by sensations of lightheadedness, dizziness, and fainting.

3. *Nausea or vomiting*: Nausea, indigestion, or vomiting may be symptoms of a heart attack, especially in women.

4. *Cold sweats*: Even if the person is not physically active, they may experience profuse perspiration, clammy skin, or cold sweats during a heart attack.

5. *Weariness or weakness*: Unexplained weariness, weakness, or excessive exhaustion may develop in the days or weeks preceding a heart attack, especially in women.

These signs and symptoms must be recognized and taken seriously, since immediate medical intervention is vital for limiting cardiac damage and improving outcomes. If you or someone else is suffering signs of a heart attack, contact 911 immediately for help. Time is of the importance when treating a heart attack, and every minute matters in terms of maintaining heart function and preventing further damage. When phoning emergency services, provide them as much information as possible about the person's symptoms, medical history, and present status so that they can respond promptly and effectively. While waiting for emergency services to come, it is critical to stay cool and soothe the affected person. Encourage them to relax in a comfortable posture and refrain from any extra exertion or activities. If the patient is aware and able to swallow, you can give them a tiny amount of aspirin (chewed or crushed) to help prevent blood clots from developing.

While waiting for emergency medical aid, there are numerous comfort measures and supportive care strategies that can help ease symptoms and reassure the affected individual:

1. *Assist with medicine*: If the client is taking medication for chest discomfort or cardiac problems, assist them in taking it as advised by their healthcare professional. Follow any particular directions issued by emergency services or medical staff.

2. *Keep the individual quiet*: Anxiety and stress can increase heart attack symptoms, therefore it's critical to keep the affected person as calm and relaxed as possible. Provide reassurance, comfort, and support, and urge them to concentrate on their breathing while remaining as motionless as possible.

3. *Monitor vital signs*: Pay particular attention to the person's pulse, respiration rate, and degree of awareness.

Prepare to do CPR or other lifesaving actions if the individual's health worsens or they become unresponsive.

4. ***Stay with the individual***: Stay with the affected person until emergency medical help comes, and then offer continuous support and assistance as required. Reassure them that aid is on its way and that they are not alone in this terrifying situation.

Providing comfort measures and supportive care while waiting for emergency medical aid might help ease symptoms and reassure the affected individual during a heart attack. Identifying and reacting quickly to the signs and symptoms of a heart attack is critical for reducing heart damage and improving outcomes. Understanding the signs of a heart attack, calling emergency services right away, and providing comfort measures and supportive care to the affected individual can help you become a critical first responder, saving lives and ensuring the best possible outcome for those suffering from a heart attack.

Shock: A Comprehensive Guide to Understanding and Managing Critical Situations

Shock is a life-threatening medical condition that occurs when the body's organs and tissues do not receive enough oxygen and nutrients due to inadequate blood flow. Shock can manifest in various ways depending on its underlying cause and severity. However, there are several common signs and symptoms that may indicate the presence of shock, including:

1. *Rapid, weak pulse*: A rapid heart rate (tachycardia) and weak pulse may indicate that the heart is working harder to compensate for decreased blood flow to the body's tissues.

2. *Pale, clammy skin*: Shock often causes the skin to become pale, cool, and clammy as the body redirects blood flow away from the skin's surface to vital organs such as the heart and brain.

3. *Rapid, shallow breathing*: Shock may lead to rapid, shallow breathing (tachypnea) as the body attempts to increase oxygen intake to compensate for decreased oxygen delivery to the tissues.

4. *Confusion or altered mental status*: In severe cases of shock, individuals may experience confusion, dizziness, fainting, or loss of consciousness due to inadequate blood flow to the brain.

5. *Low blood pressure*: Hypotension, or low blood pressure, is a common characteristic of shock and may be accompanied by other signs of cardiovascular instability, such as dizziness or lightheadedness.

It's essential to recognize these signs and symptoms promptly and take immediate action to address the underlying cause of shock and restore adequate blood flow to the body's tissues.

The primary goal of treating shock is to restore and maintain adequate blood flow to the body's organs and tissues. Depending on the underlying cause of shock, treatment may involve:

1. *Fluid resuscitation*: Administering intravenous fluids (such as saline or lactated Ringer's solution) is often the first step in treating shock to help increase blood volume and improve circulation. Fluid resuscitation should be guided by the individual's vital signs, such as blood pressure, heart rate, and urine output.

2. *Oxygen therapy*: Supplemental oxygen may be administered to individuals experiencing shock to increase oxygen delivery to the body's tissues and organs. Oxygen therapy may be provided via nasal cannula, face mask, or other delivery devices as needed.

3. *Medications*: In some cases, medications such as vasopressors or inotropes may be administered to help increase blood pressure and improve cardiac output in individuals with severe shock. These medications should be administered under the direction of a healthcare provider and monitored closely for potential side effects.

4. *Treating the underlying cause*: Identifying and addressing the underlying cause of shock is essential for effective treatment. Common causes of shock include severe bleeding (hemorrhagic shock), severe infections

(septic shock), allergic reactions (anaphylactic shock), and heart failure (cardiogenic shock).

It's essential to initiate treatment for shock promptly and continue monitoring the individual's vital signs closely to assess their response to treatment and adjust interventions as needed. While treating shock, it's crucial to monitor the individual's vital signs closely and provide reassurance and support to help alleviate anxiety and stress. Vital signs to monitor may include:

1. *Heart rate*: Monitor the individual's heart rate regularly to assess their cardiovascular status and response to treatment. A rapid or irregular heart rate may indicate ongoing shock or complications.

2. *Blood pressure*: Measure the individual's blood pressure frequently to assess their circulation and response to fluid resuscitation. Hypotension (low blood pressure) may indicate ongoing shock or inadequate perfusion to vital organs.

3. *Respiratory rate*: Monitor the individual's respiratory rate and effort to assess their oxygenation and respiratory

function. Rapid, shallow breathing may indicate respiratory distress or inadequate oxygen delivery.

4. ***Mental status***: Assess the individual's level of consciousness, orientation, and responsiveness regularly to monitor for changes in mental status. Confusion, agitation, or lethargy may indicate ongoing shock or cerebral hypoperfusion.

In addition to monitoring vital signs, it's essential to provide reassurance and support to the affected individual and their loved ones during the treatment of shock. Encourage them to remain calm and reassure them that they are receiving the necessary care and support to stabilize their condition. Shock is a life-threatening medical condition that requires prompt recognition and intervention to restore and maintain adequate blood flow to the body's organs and tissues. By understanding the signs and symptoms of shock, initiating appropriate treatment to keep blood flowing, and monitoring vital signs while providing reassurance and support, you can become a crucial first responder, helping to stabilize individuals in critical situations and improve their chances of survival.

Effective communication and coordination with emergency medical services (EMS) personnel are crucial for ensuring seamless care and transportation of injured individuals to medical facilities.

Additional Resources and Training Opportunities: Enhancing Your First Aid Skills

In addition to the valuable information provided in this handbook, there are numerous resources and training opportunities available to further enhance your first aid skills and preparedness for emergency situations. First aid certification programs offer comprehensive training in essential first aid techniques and procedures, including cardiopulmonary resuscitation (CPR), automated external defibrillator (AED) use, basic wound care, and emergency response protocols. These programs are typically offered by organizations such as the American Red Cross, the American Heart Association, and other reputable providers of first aid training. Certification courses may vary in length and content, ranging from basic courses designed for laypersons to more advanced courses tailored for healthcare professionals.

Benefits of first aid certification programs include:

1. *Comprehensive training*: Certification programs provide thorough instruction in essential first aid skills and techniques, ensuring that participants are well-prepared to respond effectively to a wide range of emergency situations.

2. *Hands-on practice*: Certification programs typically include hands-on practice sessions where participants can apply their skills in simulated emergency scenarios, helping to reinforce learning and build confidence in their abilities.

3. *Certification credentials*: Upon successful completion of a certification program, participants receive a certification card or certificate verifying their completion of the course. Certification credentials are often required or preferred for certain professions, such as childcare providers, lifeguards, and healthcare workers.

4. *Continuing education opportunities*: Many certification programs offer opportunities for ongoing education and recertification to ensure that participants stay up-to-date on the latest first aid protocols and guidelines.

Community training workshops provide valuable opportunities for individuals to learn basic first aid skills in a hands-on, interactive setting. These workshops are often offered by local organizations, such as fire departments, hospitals, schools, and community centers, and may cover topics such as CPR, AED use, choking relief, and basic wound care. Community training workshops are typically open to the public and may be offered free of charge or for a nominal fee.

Benefits of community training workshops include:

1. *Accessibility*: Community training workshops are often readily available and accessible to individuals of all ages and backgrounds, making it easy for community members to learn life-saving skills close to home.

2. *Interactive learning*: Workshops provide hands-on opportunities for participants to practice first aid skills under the guidance of trained instructors, helping to build confidence and proficiency in emergency response techniques.

3. *Community engagement*: Participating in community training workshops fosters a sense of community engagement and empowerment, as individuals come together to learn how to support and assist one another in times of need.

4. *Networking opportunities*: Workshops provide opportunities for participants to connect with other members of their community who share an interest in first aid and emergency preparedness, creating a network of support and collaboration.

In addition to formal training programs and community workshops, there is a wealth of online resources available for individuals seeking to expand their knowledge and skills in first aid and emergency response. These resources may include educational websites, instructional videos, interactive simulations, and virtual training courses covering a wide range of topics related to first aid, CPR, AED use, wilderness medicine, and more.

Benefits of online resources for ongoing education include:

1. *Flexibility and convenience*: Online resources can be accessed anytime, anywhere, allowing individuals to learn at their own pace and on their own schedule. This flexibility makes it easy to fit learning into busy lifestyles and accommodate diverse learning preferences.

2. *Variety of content*: Online resources offer a diverse array of content formats, including articles, videos, quizzes, and interactive simulations, allowing individuals to explore different learning materials and approaches to suit their preferences.

3. *Accessibility*: Online resources are often readily accessible to individuals with internet access, making them particularly valuable for individuals in remote or underserved areas where in-person training opportunities may be limited.

4. *Cost-effectiveness*: Many online resources for first aid education are available free of charge or at a low cost, making them a cost-effective option for individuals seeking to expand their knowledge and skills without breaking the bank.

In conclusion, there are numerous resources and training opportunities available to individuals seeking to enhance their first aid skills and preparedness for emergency situations. Whether through formal certification programs, community training workshops, or online resources for ongoing education, individuals can continue to build their confidence and competence as first responders, ensuring that they are well-equipped to handle a wide range of emergencies effectively. By taking advantage of these resources, you can make a meaningful difference in the lives of others and contribute to a safer and more resilient community.

First aid training courses are available for individuals of all ages and backgrounds, providing practical instruction on responding to a wide range of medical emergencies.

Special Bonus

Gain access to all my previous and future books

If you need help or questions about the first aid communities and certification programs, kindly mail to phelliprichmond92@gmail.com

Please consider writing a review!

9 798324 105709